AF431940

Table of Contents

When shopping at the grocery store, the foods you grab can greatly impact your overall health. In fact, filling your cart with a lot of refined grains, sugary drinks, and processed foods can increase inflammation and affect your health.

Therefore, filling up on healthy foods can help keep you healthy, protect against chronic diseases resistant to drugs and rid your body of toxins.

We also absorb tons of toxins every day through the air we breathe, the water we drink, the food we eat, and by just being outside in our surroundings.

So how do we get rid of these toxins that can be harmful to our body? It's through the Healing diet.

The Healing foods diet is not just a diet; It is a tool that will lead you to a total transformation of your health. This diet was designed to help everyone overcome diseases. It is designed to heal your body and improve your health by encouraging the consumption of nutritious, whole foods like fruits, veggies, legumes, healthy fats, organic meats, and healing herbs and spices.

Plus, this simple eating pattern is a great way to ensure you supply your body with a steady stream of the nutrients you need to help prevent nutritional deficiencies in your diet and to promote healthy living.

So what makes this diet unique?

This diet is unique because it involves making some simple switches in your diet compared to other complicated diets with many rules and regulations.

1. Collagen-Rich Butternut Squash Soup for Back Pain

Prep: 10 mins

Cook: 25 mins

Total: 35 mins

Servings: 6

Ingredients

- 1 butternut squash (about 1 ½ pound), peeled, seeded and cut into ½-inch cubes
- 2 tbsp olive oil
- 1 tbsp unsalted butter
- 1 medium onion, chopped
- 2 cloves garlic, minced
- ½ tsp Chinese five-spice powder
- ½ tsp ground ginger
- ½ tsp ground turmeric
- 5 cups bone broth
- salt and freshly ground pepper to taste

Directions

1. In a large pot heat the olive oil and butter over medium heat.
2. Add the onion and cook for 3-5 minutes or until softened and translucent.
3. Add the garlic and cook for 30 seconds.
4. Add the butternut squash, ground ginger, turmeric and 5 spice powder and saute for 2 minutes.
5. Add the bone broth and bring the soup to a low boil.
6. Cover with a lid and cook for 15-20 minutes or until the butternut squash is fork tender.
7. Using an immersion blender or food processor or blender, puree the soup until smooth.
8. Season to taste with salt and black pepper.
9. Serve, garnished with sour cream.

Prep: 10 mins

Cook: 20 mins

Total: 30 mins

Servings: 6

Ingredients

- medium white onion, diced (approx. 2 cups, 300 g)
- 3 carrots, chopped into thick rounds (approx. 2 cups, 300 g)
- 3 cloves garlic, minced
- 3 stalks celery, chopped (approx. 320 g)
- 1 tbsp curry powder
- 1 tsp each cumin and coriander
- 1/2 tsp each salt and pepper
- 1 1/2 cups uncooked red lentils
- 1 14 oz can light coconut milk
- 1 28 oz can diced tomatoes with the juices

- 4 cups vegetable stock
- 1 tbsp soy sauce or gluten-free tamari
- 1 tsp coconut sugar or pure maple syrup

Directions

1. Add the carrots, celery, onion and garlic to a soup pot with 2 tbsp water or broth. Cook over medium heat, stirring often, for 5-6 minutes.
2. Add the spices and stir to combine. Cook for another minute or two, adding 1-2 tbsp more water or broth if the pot is getting too dry.
3. Add the lentils, diced tomatoes, coconut milk and broth and stir to combine.
4. Simmer for 20-25 minutes, uncovered over low to medium heat until the lentils are soft and almost mushy.
5. Stir in the coconut sugar and soy sauce (or gluten-free tamari).
6. Serve right away topped with fresh cilantro, if desired.

3. Walnut Crusted Salmon

Prep: 15 mins

Cook: 33 mins

Total: 48 mins

Servings: 4

Ingredients

- 1 large sweet potato, cut into 1/2- to 1-inch cubes
- 1 large apple, cut into similar size cubes as sweet potatoes
- 1 pound Brussels sprouts, trimmed and cut in half
- 6-8 shallots, ends trimmed off, peeled and cut in half (or about the same size as the potatoes)
- 1 pound salmon
- 2/3 cup finely chopped California Walnuts
- 2 tablespoons coarse ground mustard
- 3 tablespoons real maple syrup
- 2 tablespoons olive oil, divided
- 1/2 teaspoon paprika

- 1/4 teaspoon salt more to taste
- 1/4 teaspoon black pepper more to taste

Directions

1. Preheat oven to 425°F.
2. Line a rimmed baking sheet with parchment paper.
3. Toss sweet potatoes, Brussels sprouts, and shallots with 1 tablespoon olive oil (I sometimes do it in a zip-top bag!). Spread on sheet pan and sprinkle with salt and pepper as desired.
4. Place in oven and cook for 15 minutes.
5. Meanwhile, rinse salmon and pat dry. Prepare walnut mixture in a small bowl, stirring together walnuts, mustard, maple syrup, 1 tablespoon olive oil, paprika, salt and pepper.
6. After 15 minutes, toss vegetables around and push them to the edges of the pan to make room for the salmon.

7. Place salmon on pan and spoon walnut mixture on top. Sprinkle apples around the salmon with the vegetables.

8. Return to oven and cook for 15-18 minutes or until fish is flaky or reaches an internal temperature at its thickest portion of 145°F.

Prep: 15 mins

Cook: 20 mins

Total: 35 mins

Servings: 1

Ingredients

- 2.5 oz herb salad mix (mix of baby lettuces, red & green chard, mizuna, arugula, friseé, radicchio, parsley, cilantro, dill, baby spinach)
- 1 tablespoon coconut oil, melted
- ½ tablespoon maple syrup
- ½ tablespoon lemon juice
- coconut oil, for cooking
- ½ cup apples, thinly sliced
- ½ cup grapes, chopped
- handful walnuts, chopped

Directions

1. Tear salad leaves into bite-sized pieces.
2. Combine coconut oil, maple syrup, and lemon juice in small bowl. Pour over salad and massage gently onto the leaves.
3. Heat a skillet on medium heat and place aprox. ½ tablespoon coconut oil in it.
4. Place slices of apple in pan.
5. Sprinkle with cinnamon. Drizzle with maple syrup (optional).
6. When they begin to become golden brown and become soft, flip and pan-fry the other sides until golden brown.
7. Turn off heat and add apples to your salad bowl.
8. Place the chopped grapes into the pan, just to let them become a luke-warm temperature.
9. Combine grapes in salad.
10. Top with chopped walnuts. Enjoy!

Prep: 20 mins

Total: 20 mins

Servings: 15

Ingredients

- 1 cup peanut butter or any other nut butter for Paleo
- 4 tbsp. vanilla protein powder
- 2 tbsp. Gluten Free Oat Flour or coconut flour
- 2 tbsp. unsweetened almond milk
- 1 tbsp. unsweetened applesauce
- 1/2 tsp. cinnamon
- 2 tsp. turmeric
- 3 tbsp. unsweetened coconut flakes for rolling

Directions

1. In a mixing bowl, combine all ingredients omitting the shredded coconut flakes. Stir to

combine. You can also use a blender or food processor!

2. Once combined, place two plates on the counter. One with the shredded coconut flakes. Another for set the bites on.

3. Scoop a tablespoon of batter and roll into balls. Wetting your hands will help to make the balls stick together and roll easier!

4. Roll the ball over the shredded coconut flakes then place on the empty plate. Repeat until the batter is complete.

5. Place in the refrigerator 20-30 minutes to harden and enjoy!

Prep: 10 mins

Total: 10 mins

Servings: 4

Ingredients

- 2 tablespoons extra-virgin olive oil
- 2 tablespoons fresh lemon juice
- 1 tablespoon chopped fresh oregano
- 4 cups (packed) baby spinach leaves, coarsely chopped (about 4 ounces)
- 1 1/2 large red bell peppers, diced
- 1 1/2 cups diced celery (about 3 stalks)
- 3/4 cup crumbled soft fresh goat cheese
- 1/3 cup chopped red onion

Directions

1. Whisk oil, lemon juice, and oregano in large bowl to blend.

2. Season to taste with salt and pepper. Add spinach, bell peppers, celery, goat cheese, and red onion to dressing; toss to coat.

3. Divide salad among 4 plates and serve.

Prep: 10 mins

Total: 10 mins

Servings: 2

Ingredients

- 8-10 carrots
- 6 clementines, peeled
- 1-inch ginger
- 4 pieces fresh turmeric (or 1/2 teaspoon ground turmeric)

Directions

1. Scrub the carrots well to remove any dirt, trim the tops of the carrots. Remove the peels from the clementines.
2. Process all ingredients through your juicer.
3. If using ground turmeric, pour juice into a glass and stir in the turmeric until well combined.

4. Stir in the essential oil.

5. Enjoy within 30 minutes of juicing or pour into an airtight container to store in your refrigerator for up 36 hours.

Prep: 10 mins

Cook: 20 mins

Total: 30 mins

Servings: 4

Ingredients

Vegetables:

- 16 ounces peeled carrots, cut into 1/2" dice to equal about 3 cups
- 8 ounces lightly peeled parsnips, cut into 1/2" dice to equal about 1 1/2 cups
- 8 ounces red potatoes (NOT peeled), cut into 1/2" dice to equal about 1 1/2 cups
- 4 teaspoons extra virgin olive oil
- 1/2 teaspoon kosher salt
- 1/4 teaspoon black pepper

Drizzle:

- 1 1/2 tablespoons apple cider vinegar
- 1 tablespoon extra virgin olive oil
- 1 tablespoon honey
- 1 tablespoon smooth dijon mustard
- 1/16 teaspoon kosher salt
- optional: chopped parsley for garnish

Directions

1. Preheat oven to 475°F. Line a large baking sheet with parchment paper.
2. Toss vegetables with 4 teaspoons oil, 1/2 teaspoon salt, and 1/4 teaspoon black pepper. Make sure that the vegetables are evenly coated with oil, and that the seasonings are distributed throughout. (You can do this in a bowl, or directly on the parchment-lined baking sheet.)
3. Spread the vegetables out on the baking sheet so they aren't piled on top of each other. (If you have a smaller baking sheet and the vegetables are

crowded, it's best to grab a second baking sheet, rather than piling the veggies up.)

4. Roast the vegetables for about 12 minutes. Stir vegetables and continue roasting for 8-10 minutes longer, until the vegetables have toasty, browned, roasted spots but aren't burned.

5. While the vegetables are roasting, whisk together all ingredients for the Honey-Dijon Drizzle (vinegar, olive oil, honey, mustard, and salt).

6. Serve vegetables warm, drizzled with Honey-Dijon sauce and sprinkled with a little chopped fresh parsley, if desired.

Prep: 3 mins

Cook: 3 mins

Additional: 4 mins

Total: 10 mins

Servings: 1

Ingredients

- 1 cup unsweetened almond or rice milk
- 1/3 cup quinoa flakes
- 1/4 cup pomegranate seeds
- 1 pinch sea salt
- maple syrup or raw honey optional, to sweeten
- toasted walnuts, almonds, granola or berries, optional

Directions

1. In a small or medium saucepan set to medium-high heat, bring the milk to a boil.

2. Once the milk comes to a boil, add the quinoa flakes, pomegranate seeds and a pinch of salt. Turn off the heat and stir a few times.

3. Allow cereal to sit for 3 minutes. Stir cereal one last time to make it thicker.

4. Scoop cereal into bowl and drizzle with maple syrup or honey. Add desired toppings.

Prep: 20 mins

Cook: 20 mins

Total: 40 mins

Servings: 4

Ingredients

- 1 tsp. ground cumin
- 1/2 tsp. garlic powder
- 1/4 tsp. chipotle chili powder
- kosher salt
- Pepper
- 1 tbsp. olive oil
- 2 large boneless, skinless chicken breasts
- 4 medium radishes
- 2 scallions
- 1 large avocado
- 1/4 c. pomegranate seeds

- 1 tbsp. fresh lime juice
- 1/2 c. fresh cilantro leaves
- 8 small flour tortillas
- sour cream

Directions

1. Heat oven to 425 degrees F. Line a rimmed baking sheet with foil. In a small bowl, combine the cumin, garlic, chili powders, and 1/2 teaspoon salt.
2. Heat the oil in a medium skillet over medium heat. Season the chicken with the spice mixture and cook until browned, 2 to 3 minutes per side. Transfer the chicken to the baking sheet and roast until cooked through, 8 to 10 minutes.
3. Meanwhile, in a medium bowl, gently toss together the radishes, scallions, avocado, pomegranate seeds, lime juice, and 1/4 teaspoon each salt and pepper; fold in the cilantro.
4. Slice the chicken into 1/4-inch-thick pieces. Fill the tortillas with the chicken and top with the

pomegranate salsa. Serve with sour cream, if desired.

Prep: 5 mins

Total: 5 mins

Servings: 1

Ingredients

- 3/4 cup almond milk
- 1/2 tablespoon coconut butter
- 2 dates, pitted
- 1/2-1 teaspoon turmeric
- 1/4 teaspoon cinnamon
- 1/4 teaspoon ginger
- pinch ground pepper
- 1 cup ice

Directions

1. Add all ingredients to a high-speed blender.
2. Blend on high until smooth.
3. Pour into glass and top with dairy-free whipped cream and cinnamon, if desired.

Prep: 10 mins

Total: 10 mins

Servings: 1

Ingredients

- 2 cups shelled edamame
- 1/2 cup chopped red onion
- juice of 1 lime
- sea salt
- handful of cilantro
- diced tomatoes (optional)
- chili flakes (optional)

Preparation

1. Simply pulse the onion in a blender for a few seconds. Then add the rest of the ingredients and pulse until the edamame is blended into big chunks.

2. Enjoy as a spread on toast, for a sandwich, as a
    dip or as a pesto sauce!

Prep: 40 mins

Total: 40 mins

Servings: 6

Ingredients

White Chocolate Layer:

- 1 cup cashews, soaked in water
- 2/3 cup coconut water
- 1/2 cup pitted Medjool dates
- 1/4 cup cacao butter, melted
- Juice of 1 lemon
- 1 teaspoon vanilla extract
- Pinch of sea salt

Mocha Layer:

- 1 cup cashews, soaked in water
- 1/3 cup maple syrup
- 1/4 cup coconut water

- 1/4 cup brewed espresso, chilled
- 1/4 cup cacao powder
- Pinch of sea salt

Directions

1. Blend all of the ingredients for the white chocolate layer in a high speed blender or food processor until smooth.
2. Blend all of the ingredients for the mocha layer in a high speed blender or food processor until smooth.
3. Layer the white chocolate and the mocha layers in jars and refrigerate them for a few hours, or freeze for 30 to 40 minutes before serving.

Prep: 30 mins

Bake: 1 hr 10 mins

Total: 1 hr 40 mins

Servings: 4

Ingredients

Dry:

- 1-1/2 cups gluten-free baking flour
- 1/4 teaspoon salt
- 1 teaspoon baking soda
- 1/4 teaspoon pure stevia extract powder
- 1 cup fresh red grapes, halved

Wet:

- 1-1/2 teaspoons vegan egg replacer of your choice
- 2 teaspoons water
- 1 cup unsweetened applesauce
- 1/4 cup olive oil

- 1/2 tablespoon white distilled vinegar

- 1/2 cup soy milk

- 2 teaspoons vegan butter (for greasing the springform pan)

Grape Syrup and Garnishing:

- 3 cups grape juice (100 percent, no sugar added)

- 1/2 teaspoon organic powdered sugar, optional

Directions

1. Preheat the oven to 350 °F. Butter the springform pan. In a large mixing bowl, whisk all the dry ingredients together except the grapes. Set aside. In another mixing bowl, whisk together the egg replacer and water. Let it stand at room temperature for 2 minutes. Mix in the remaining wet ingredients.

2. Pour the wet ingredients mixture into the dry ingredient mixture. Mix until just combined. Fold 3/4 cup grapes in the flour mixture. Scrape the

batter into the prepared springform pan. Arrange the remaining grapes on top of the batter.

3. Bake for 35 minutes until a cake tester (such as a toothpick) inserted in the center comes out clean. Place the pan onto a cooling rack and let it stand for five minutes before removing the ring. Let it cool.

4. While the cake is baking, boil grape juice in a saucepan over high heat until reduced to 1/3 cup. Approximately 40 minutes.

5. Remove the cake from the base and transfer it onto a serving platter. Dust the top of the cake with powdered sugar before serving. Serve with the grape syrup at the table.

Prep: 10 mins

Cook: 10 mins

Total: 20 mins

Servings: 4

Ingredients

- 2 tablespoons ground nut oil
- 2 cloves garlic, minced
- 1 thumb sized piece of ginger, minced
- 2 dried chillies, chopped (optional)
- 3 cups mushrooms, sliced
- 1 cup frozen and thawed edamame (soya beans)
- 1 cup bamboo shoots, sliced
- 2 tablespoons soya sauce

Directions

1. Heat the oil in a wok and add the garlic, ginger and chillies, if using, and stir fry until fragrant.
2. Add the mushrooms and cook until soft.

3. Add the edamame, bamboo shoots and soya sauce
    and cook for 5 minutes.
4. Serve over rice, noodles or on its own.

Prep: 5 mins

Total: 5 mins

Servings: 2

Ingredients

- 1/2 cup almond milk
- 1/2 cup coconut milk yogurt
- 1 scoop plant based protein powder, vanilla
- 1/2 frozen banana
- 1/2 cup cauliflower, steamed then frozen
- 1/2 teaspoon turmeric
- 1/2 teaspoon cinnamon
- 1/4 teaspoon ginger
- Blueberries
- Blackberries
- Chopped almonds
- Hemp Seeds

Directions

1. Place smoothie ingredients into a high-speed blender. Blend on high until smooth.
2. Pour smoothie into a bowl. Top with desired toppings.

17. Oil-Free Baked Tofu

Prep: 10 mins

Cook: 30 mins

Total: 40 mins

Servings: 4

Ingredients

- 16- ounce package of extra firm tofu
- 1 teaspoon of Himalayan pink salt or sea salt
- 2 tablespoons of nutritional yeast
- 2 tablespoons onion powder
- 1 tablespoon cajun seasoning
- 1 tablespoon smoked paprika
- A few pinches of cayenne pepper, optional
- 1/2 teaspoon of turmeric
- A few pinches of black pepper

Directions

- Pre-heat your oven to 400 degree F.

- Chop tofu into even-sized pieces, and place on a baking sheet. Mix with all seasonings, and bake at 400 degree F for 25-30 minutes (the tofu looks like it is slightly puffing up when it is ready).

Prep: 30 mins

Refrigerate: 18 hrs

Total: 18 hrs 30 mins

Servings: 4

Ingredients

- 1/3 cup (60 g) medium-ground coffee beans
- 2 1/2 cups (600 ml) all-natural canned coconut milk
- 1/4 cup (50 g) organic unrefined cane sugar
- 1/4 cup (60 ml) agave
- 1 tablespoon (15 ml) pure vanilla extract
- Pinch of sea salt

Directions

1. In a bowl, combine the coffee grounds and coconut milk. Cover this mixture and place it in the refrigerator to steep overnight, at least 12 hours or more.

2. Once it's steeped, use a fine-mesh strainer to remove the grounds from the coconut milk. If you find that your coconut milk has separated and there is a layer of cream on top, stir it and let the milk warm enough to homogenize before straining it. Discard the grounds.

3. Use a high-speed or immersion blender to mix the coconut milk coffee, sugar, agave, vanilla, and salt. Add the mixture to your ice cream maker and churn it according to the manufacturer's instructions. Most machines take 10 to 15 minutes depending on the temperature of the mix, and when it's finished it should look like soft serve.

4. Once it's churned, transfer the ice cream to a large freezer-safe container, smooth the top, and cover it tightly. Freeze the finished ice cream for at least 5 to 6 hours, or until it is firm. Store this ice cream in the freezer in a sealed container for up to 1 week.

Prep: 10 mins

Cook: 45 mins

Total: 55 mins

Servings: 4

Ingredients

- 4 cups grapes
- 3 teaspoons chia seeds
- 1 teaspoons stevia (optional)

Directions

1. Put the grapes in a covered pot and let them cook on a low heat for 20-30 minutes.
2. During the process stir the grapes and with a spoon or a fork to punch the berries to drop all the juice.

3. To discard the peels and the grains pass the juice through a network dowel and go crushing with a fork or a pestle to make the most of it.

4. Put the unsweetened juice in the pot again and boil it with the chia seeds for 15 minutes and if you wish to add a spoonful of stevia or another sweetener go ahead.

5. Remove from heat. If you want to go with the magic wand. Put it in a jar and let it cool. Then put it in the refrigerator and consume within 2 weeks.

Prep: 10 mins

Total: 10 mins

Servings: 1

Ingredients

Beet Ginger Juice:

- 3 medium beets, peeled and diced
- 1 (1-inch) piece peeled fresh ginger
- 1/2 cup water

Moscow Mule:

- Crushed ice, as needed
- Ice cubes, as needed
- 2 ounces vodka
- 1 1/2 ounce fresh lime juice
- 3 to 4 ounces ginger beer
- Lime wedges, as needed

Directions

1. To make the beet-ginger juice, combine the beets, ginger, and water in a blender or food processor and blend until smooth. Strain the mixture through a fine-mesh strainer or cheesecloth into a medium bowl. Discard the pulp and set the juice aside.

2. To make the Moscow Mule, fill a mule mug or glass with crushed ice. Add a few ice cubes to a cocktail shaker. Add the vodka, lime juice, and 1 1/2 ounces of the beet-ginger juice to the shaker and shake for 20 to 30 seconds.

3. Pour the mixture into the prepared glass and top with the ginger beer. Stir to combine and garnish with a lime wedge.

Prep: 10 mins

Cook: 40 mins

Total: 50 mins

Servings: 3

Ingredients

- 17 1/2 ounces brussels sprouts
- 6 tablespoons extra virgin olive oil
- Salt
- Pepper
- Red chili flakes
- Turmeric
- 1 tablespoon vegan butter (optional)
- Baby spinach leaves for decorations
- Cumin

Directions

1. Preheat oven to 390°F. Trim bottom of Brussels sprouts and cut them in half. Mix the sprouts in a bowl with the condiments, olive oil and vegan butter.

2. Put them in a covered baking tray for 35 to 40 minutes, until crisp on the outside and tender on the inside. Taste, and add more salt and pepper if necessary. Enjoy!

Prep: 5 mins

Total: 5 mins

Servings: 2

Ingredients

- 1 cup almond milk
- 1 strong espresso

Directions

1. Pour the almond milk in a glass and dip the steamer pipe in the milk no more than half an inch
2. Warm the milk and keep on turning the glass until you have thick milk foam. Do not let the milk cook.
3. Make a strong espresso and pour it into the milk

Prep: 5 mins

Cook: 5 mins

Total: 10 mins

Servings: 4

Ingredients

- 1/4 cup honey
- 1/2 cup balsamic vinegar
- 1 teaspoon salt
- 1 teaspoon red pepper flakes
- 24 large red seedless grapes
- 16 jumbo shrimps (about 1 pound), peeled and deveined
- 8 skewers
- 2 tablespoons vegetable oil

Directions

1. Combine the honey, vinegar and 1/2 teaspoon of the salt in a nonstick skillet over medium heat. Cook for 3 to 4 minutes, until bubbly and thick. Remove from the heat and stir in the red pepper flakes. Keep warm.

2. Starting and ending with a grape, alternately thread grapes (3 in total) and shrimp (2) on each skewer. Sprinkle with the remaining salt.

3. Brush a large nonstick grill pan or cast-iron skillet with 1 teaspoon of the oil. Place the pan over medium-high heat until it is very hot but not smoking. Arrange the skewers in the pan and cook, basting with the remaining oil and turning frequently, until the shrimp are cooked on all sides, about 4 minutes.

4. Transfer the skewers to a serving platter. Drizzle with the sauce and serve hot.

Prep: 5 mins

Cook: 10 mins

Total: 15 mins

Servings: 4

Ingredients

- 2 tablespoons cornstarch
- 2 tablespoons water
- 1 pound skinless, boneless chicken thighs, cut into 1/2-inch cubes
- 2 tablespoons vegetable oil
- 2 dried red chilis
- 1-inch piece ginger, peeled and minced
- 2 tablespoons honey
- 3 1/2 tablespoons soy sauce
- 2 tablespoons rice vinegar
- 1 teaspoon grated lemon zest
- 12 to 14 fresh basil leaves, chopped

- Thinly sliced, peeled ginger, for garnish

Directions

1. In a medium bowl, mix the cornstarch and water into a paste. Add the chicken pieces and toss well to coat.
2. Heat the oil in a wok or large skillet over medium-high heat until very hot. Add the chicken and stir-fry until it is cooked through and lightly browned, 4 to 5 minutes.
3. Add the chilis and minced ginger and stir-fry for another minute.
4. Stir in the honey, soy sauce and vinegar and cook for 1 minute or so, until the sauce is slightly thickened. Sprinkle with the lemon zest and heat through, about 30 seconds.
5. Transfer to a serving platter and top with the basil and sliced ginger.

Prep: 5 mins

Cook: 10 mins

Total: 15 mins

Servings: 4

Ingredients

- 1 pound skinless, boneless chicken thighs, cut crosswise into 1/2-inch-thick strips
- Salt
- Freshly ground black pepper
- 2 tablespoons peanut oil
- 1 teaspoon sugar
- 3 cloves garlic, minced
- 1/2 teaspoon Chinese five-spice powder
- 1 cup frozen shelled edamame, thawed
- 1 teaspoon grated fresh ginger
- 3 tablespoons teriyaki sauce
- 1 teaspoon sesame seeds

- 1/2 cup diced baby corn
- 2 scallions, thinly sliced on the diagonal
- 2 cups steamed white rice

Directions

1. Season the chicken lightly with salt and pepper.
2. Place a wok or large skillet over high heat and pour in the oil. As soon as the oil is hot, add the chicken and stir-fry for about 3 minutes, until the chicken is almost cooked through.
3. Add the sugar, garlic, five-spice powder, edamame and ginger, and stir-fry for 3 minutes more, stirring constantly so the garlic doesn't burn.
4. Add the teriyaki sauce, sesame seeds, corn and scallions. Continue to stir and toss until everything is evenly coated with the sauce and heated through. Serve hot over steamed rice.

Prep: 5 mins

Cook: 10 mins

Total: 15 mins

Servings: 4

Ingredients

- 1/4 cup extra-virgin olive oil
- 1 small head cauliflower, broken into florets
- 1 teaspoon turmeric
- Leaves from 1 sprig rosemary
- Salt and freshly ground black pepper
- 1/4 cup golden raisins
- 1/4 cup pine nuts, toasted
- 1 teaspoon smoked Spanish paprika

Directions

1. Heat the olive oil in a medium skillet over medium heat.
2. Add the cauliflower, turmeric and rosemary and cook, stirring occasionally, until the cauliflower is brown and caramelized, about 8 minutes.
3. Season with salt and pepper to taste.
4. Stir in the raisins and pine nuts and cook about 1 minute more, until everything is heated through.
5. Transfer to a serving bowl and sprinkle with paprika.

Prep: 15 mins

Total: 15 mins

Servings: 4

- 3 tablespoons light mayonnaise
- 1 1/2 teaspoons curry powder
- 2 cups cubed cooked chicken
- 1 cup fresh cherries, pitted and sliced
- 1 small ripe mango, peeled, pitted and diced
- 1/4 small red onion, diced
- 2 tablespoons minced cilantro
- Salt
- Freshly ground black pepper
- 1/2 cup chopped roasted pecans

Directions

1. In a large bowl, mix the mayonnaise and the curry powder.

2. Fold in the chicken, cherries, mango, onion and cilantro. Season to taste with salt and pepper.

3. Sprinkle with the pecans and serve.

Prep: 5 mins

Total: 5 mins

Servings: 2

Ingredients

- 2 scoops low-fat coffee ice cream
- 1 cup chilled skim milk
- 1 cup cracked ice
- 1/2 teaspoon instant coffee, plus more for garnish

Directions

1. Combine all ingredients (except garnish) in a blender and blend well.
2. Pour into 2 tall glasses. Garnish with a sprinkle of instant coffee and serve immediately.

Prep: 5 mins

Cook: 5 mins

Total: 10 mins

Servings: 4

Ingredients

- 4 thin slices pancetta (about 1 ounce total)
- 1/4 cup crème fraîche
- 8 slices white or whole-wheat bread
- Freshly ground black pepper
- 1/4 medium English cucumber, very thinly sliced
- 8 to 12 small sprigs watercress, tough stems removed
- 1/4 pound thinly sliced cold smoked salmon

Directions

1. Heat a skillet over medium heat. Cook the pancetta, turning once, until well browned, about

5 minutes. Drain on paper towels. When it is cool enough to handle, break into small pieces.

2. Spread the crème fraîche generously on one side of each bread slice. Sprinkle a little black pepper on each slice.

3. Top 4 bread slices with the crumbled pancetta, cucumber, watercress and salmon. Cover with a second slice of bread. Cut each sandwich into halves or quarters, depending on your preference. Serve immediately.

Prep: 5 mins

Prep: 10 mins

Total: 10 mins

Servings: 4

Ingredients:

- 1 cup dried, unsweetened cherries (try to find the unsulfured variety), chopped coarsely
- ½ cup unsweetened shredded coconut
- 1 cup toasted almonds, chopped coarsely
- 6 oz dark chocolate chopped or 6 oz semi-sweet chocolate chips (try to find those without soy lecithin)

Directions

1. Line a baking sheet with BPA-free parchment paper, slick side-up.

2. In a medium mixing bowl, combine the cherries, almonds and coconut.

3. In the top of a double boiler, melt half of the chocolate over low-medium heat. Stir regularly, until completely melted. Remove from heat. (If you don't own a double boiler, you can melt your chocolate in the microwave. Put all chocolate in a medium microwave-safe bowl. Heat on high in 15-second increments, removing and stirring between each cycle until melted)

4. Stir the fruits and nuts into the chocolate until all ingredients are thoroughly coated.

5. Scoop out heaping tablespoons of the mixture onto lined baking sheet.

6. Once all mixture has been used, place in the fridge for about 20 minutes to set.

7. Store in an airtight container at room temperature.